Our Bodies

Our Hearts

Charlotte Guillain

Heinemann Library
Chicago, Illinois

www.heinemannraintree.com
Visit our website to find out
more information about
Heinemann-Raintree books.

To order:

☎ Phone 888-454-2279

🖳 Visit www.heinemannraintree.com
to browse our catalog and order online.

©2010 Heinemann Library
a division of Capstone Global Library LLC
Chicago, Illinois
All rights reserved. No part of this publication may be reproduced
or transmitted in any form or by any means, electronic or
mechanical, including photocopying, recording, taping, or any
information storage and retrieval system, without permission in
writing from the publisher.

Editorial: Rebecca Rissman, Laura Knowles, Nancy Dickmann,
 and Sian Smith
Picture research: Ruth Blair and Mica Brancic
Designed by Joanna Hinton-Malivoire
Original Illustrations © Capstone Global Library Ltd. 2010
Illustrated by Tony Wilson
Printed and bound by Leo Paper Group

14 13 12 11 10
10 9 8 7 6 5 4 3 2 1

Library of Congress Cataloging-in-Publication Data
Guillain, Charlotte.
 Our hearts / Charlotte Guillain.
   p. cm. -- (Our bodies)
 Includes bibliographical references and index.
 ISBN 978-1-4329-3590-0 (hc) -- ISBN 978-1-4329-3599-3 (pb)
 1. Heart--Juvenile literature. I. Title.
 QP111.6.G85 2010
 612.1'7--dc22
                        2009022294

Acknowledgments
The author and publisher are grateful to the following for
permission to reproduce copyright material:
We would like to thank the following for permission to reproduce
photographs: Corbis pp.**8** (© Stephanie Weiler/zefa), **9** (© Hannah
Mentz/zefa), **10** (© John-Francis Bourke/zefa), **17**, **18** (© moodboard),
20 (© Randy Faris); iStockphoto p.**21**; Photolibrary pp.**4**, **22** (© OJO
Images), **5** (© Photoalto), **14** (© Tips Italia), **16** (© Photoalto), **23**
(© Tips Italia); Science Photo Library pp.**11**, **23** (© Medi-Mation);
Shutterstock p.**19** (© Jacek Chabraszewski).

Front cover photograph of children jumping down a sand dune
reproduced with permission of Photolibrary (© Swell Media/Uppercut
Images). Back cover photograph reproduced with permission of
Photolibrary (Photoalto).

Every effort has been made to contact copyright holders of any
material reproduced in this book. Any omissions will be rectified in
subsequent printings if notice is given to the publisher.

Contents

Body Parts

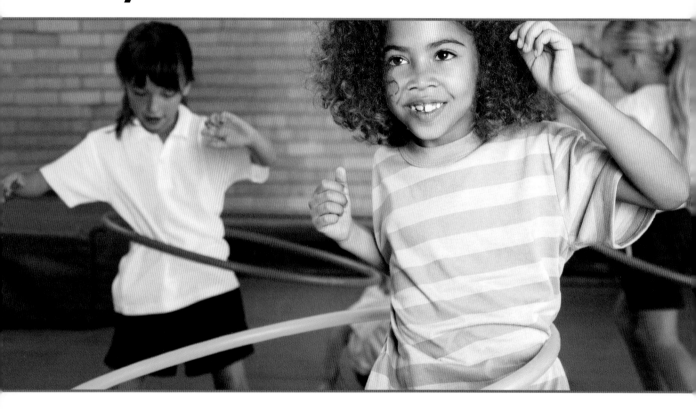

Our bodies have many parts.

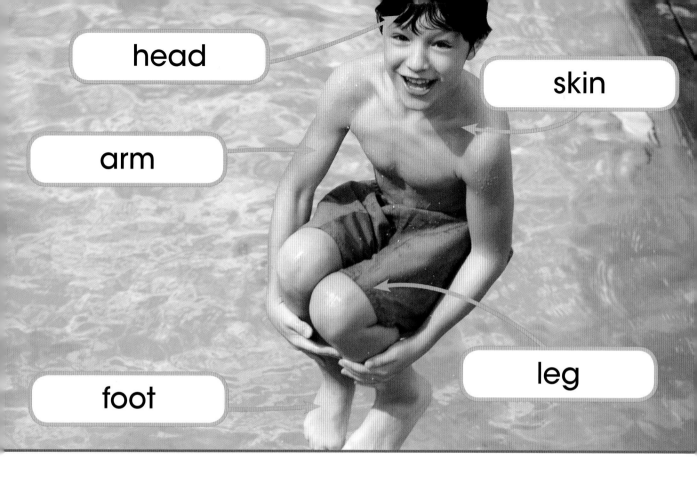

head

skin

arm

leg

foot

Our bodies have parts on
the outside.

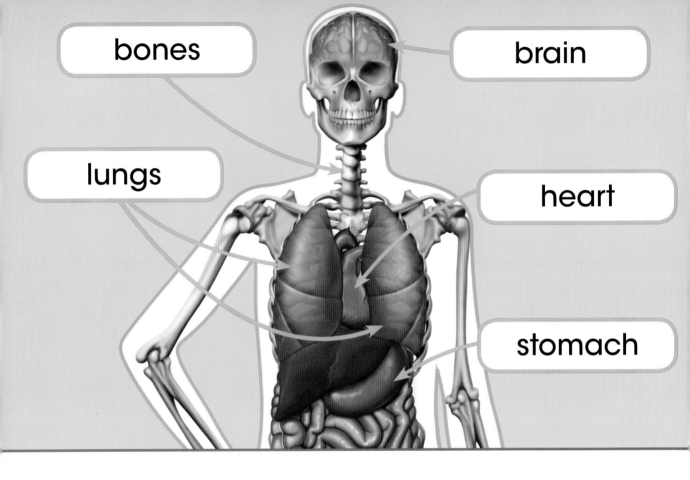

bones

brain

lungs

heart

stomach

Our bodies have parts on
the inside.

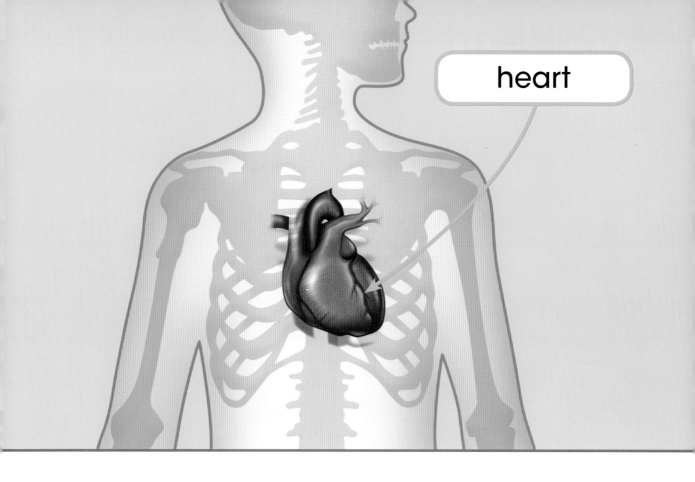

heart

Your heart is inside your body.

Your Heart

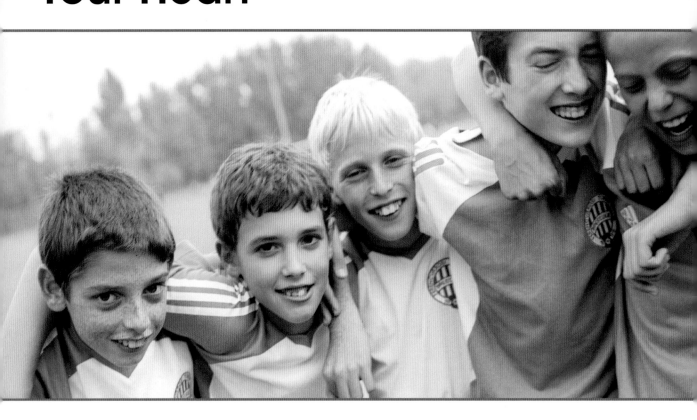

You cannot see your heart.

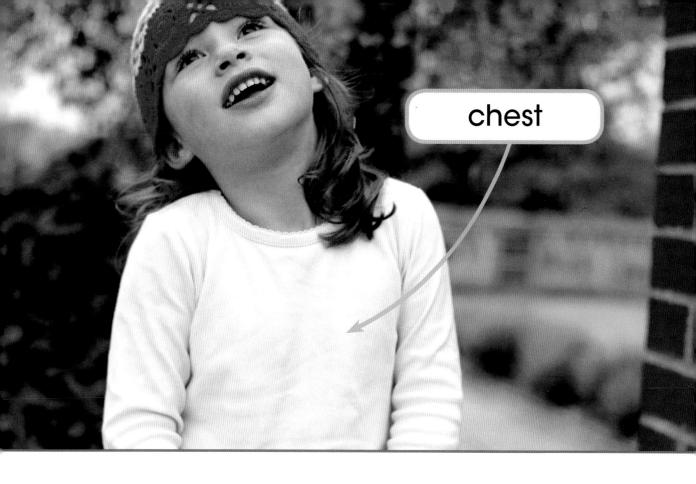

chest

Your heart is inside your chest.

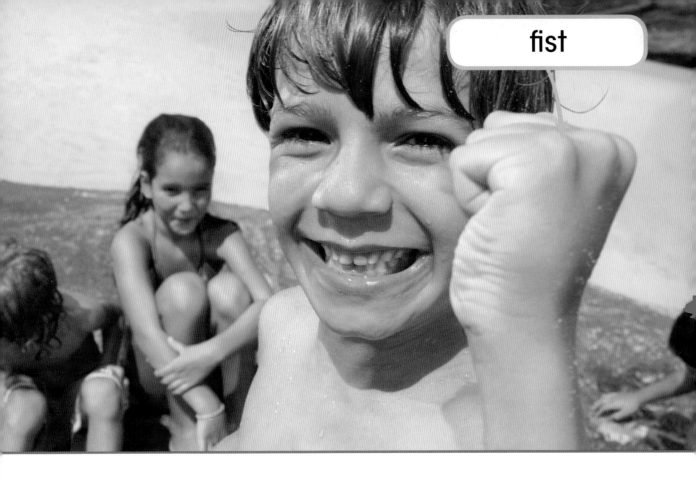

fist

Your heart is about the size of
your fist.

10

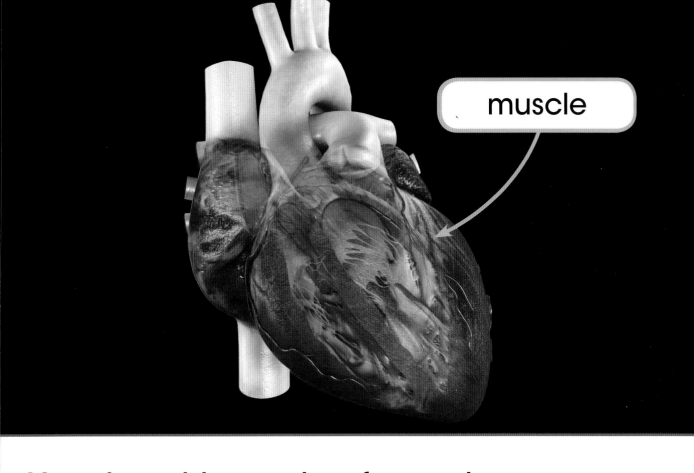

muscle

Your heart is made of muscle.

Muscles can make things move.

Blood

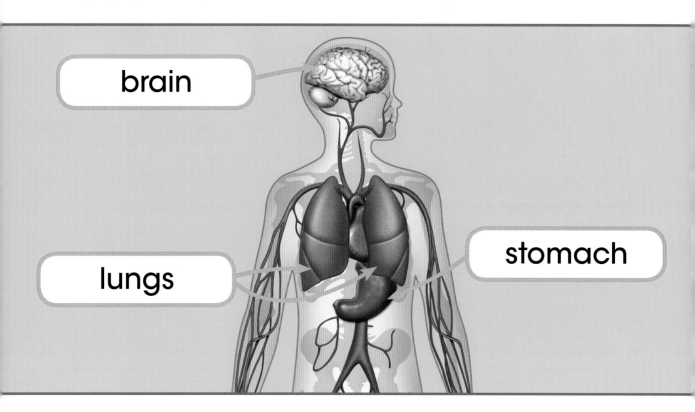

brain

lungs

stomach

Your body parts need blood.

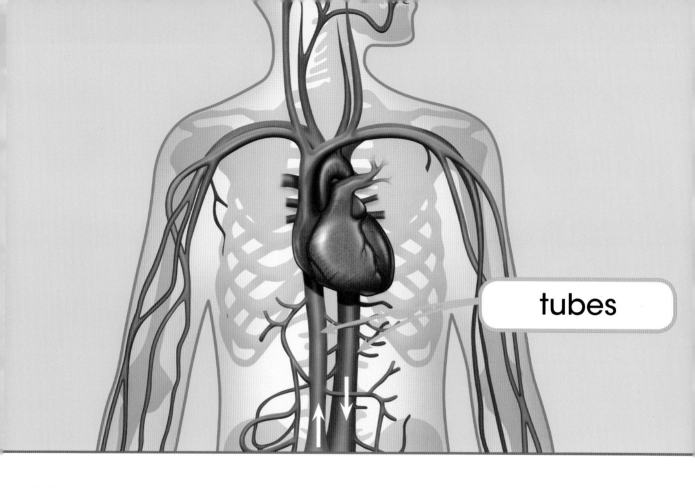

tubes

Blood moves around your body
in tubes.

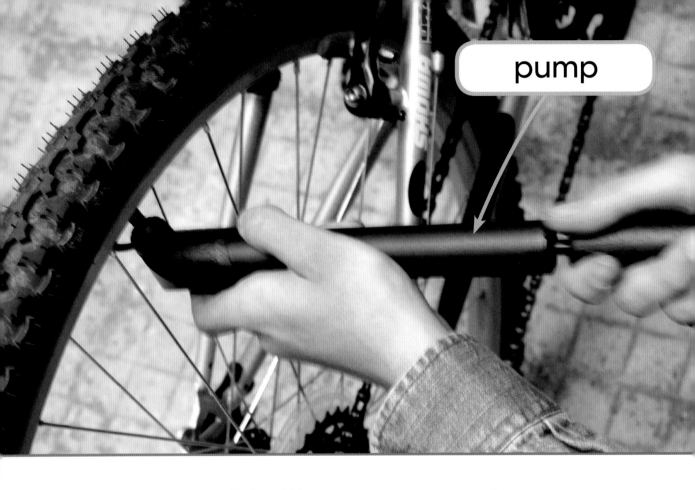

pump

Your heart is like a pump. A pump
pushes air into a tire.

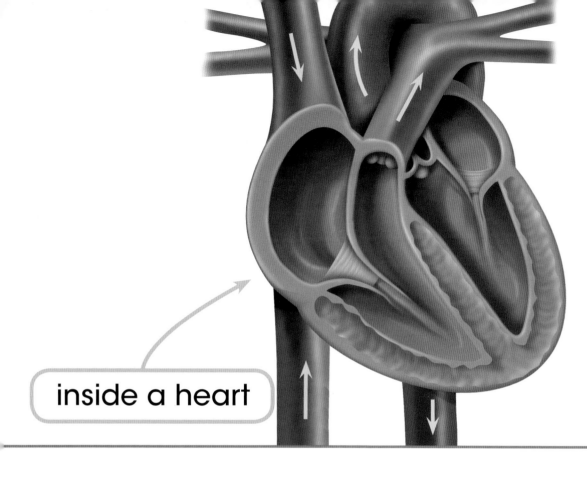

inside a heart

Your heart pushes blood around
your body.

Heart Beat

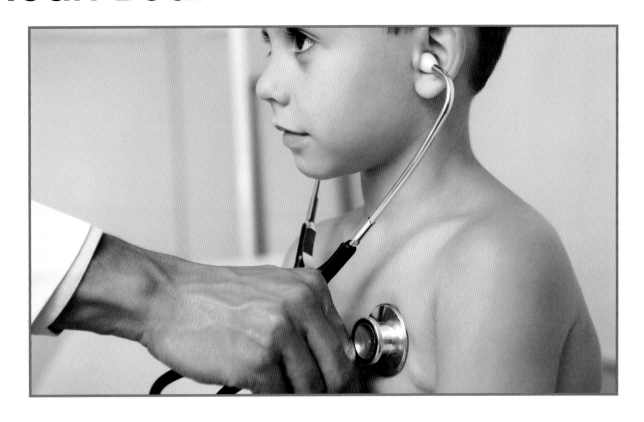

You can hear your heart beat.

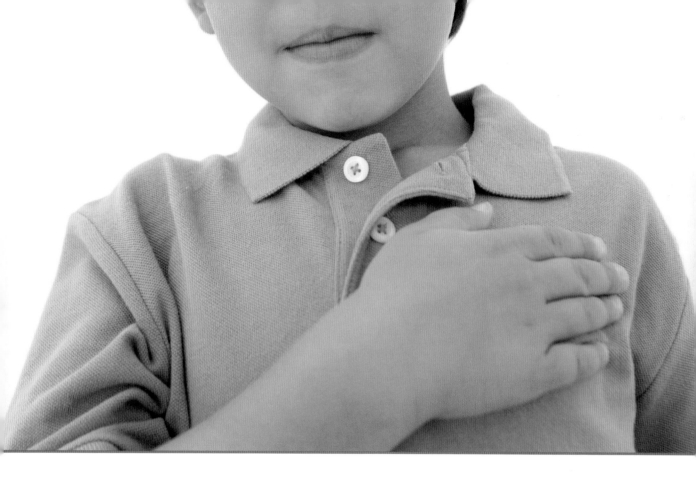

You can feel your heart beat.

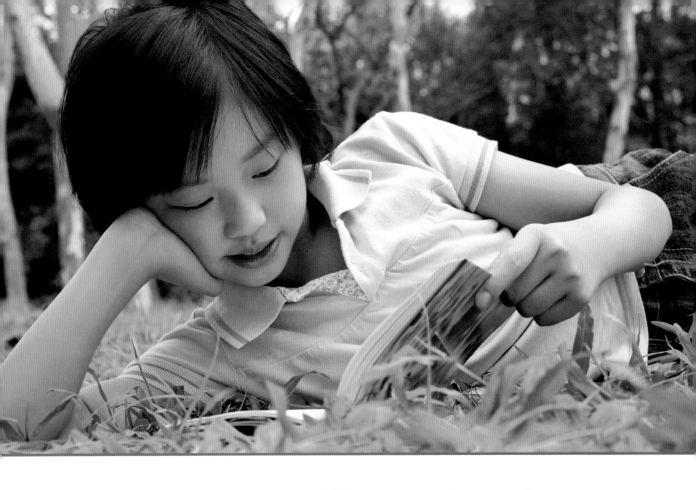

When you are still, your heart beats slowly.

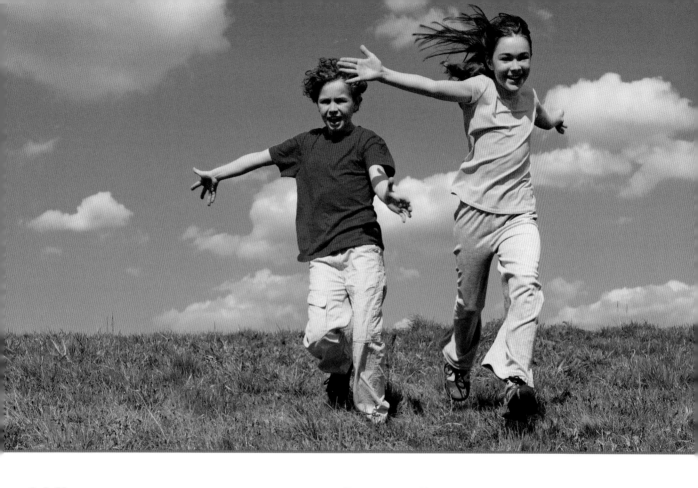

When you run, your heart
beats fast.

Staying Healthy

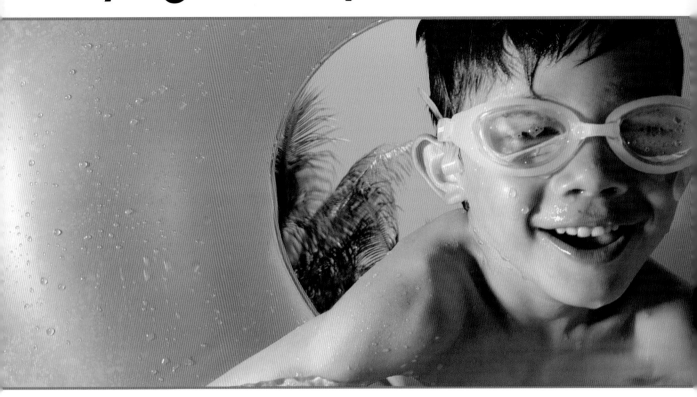

You can exercise to help your heart.

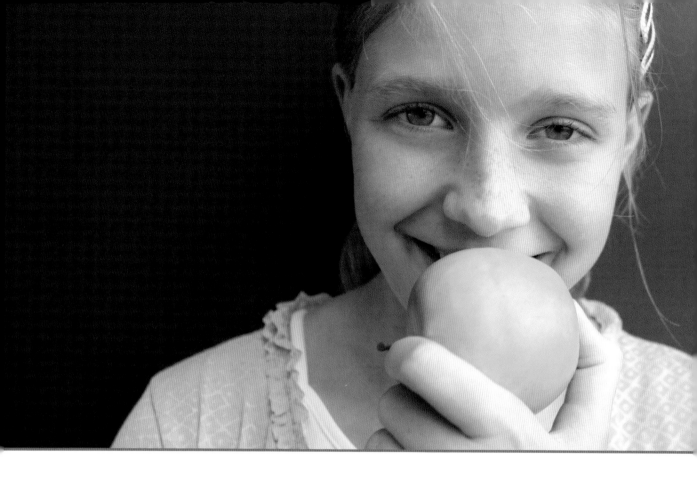

You can eat healthy food to help
your heart.

Quiz

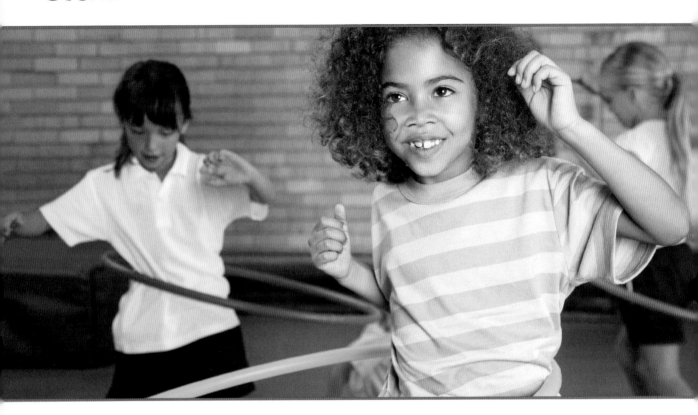

Where in your body is your heart?

Answer on page 24

Picture Glossary

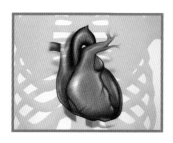 **heart** part of your body inside your chest. Your heart pushes blood around your body.

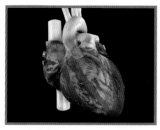 **muscle** stretchy part inside your body. Muscles can make things move.

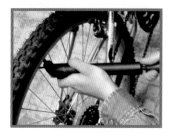 **pump** something you use to push air into a tire

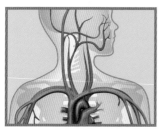 **tube** a long, thin pipe like a hose. Things can move through tubes because they have an empty space in the middle.

Index

Answer to quiz on page 22: Your heart is in your chest.

Notes to parents and teachers

Before reading

Ask children to name the parts of their body they can see on the outside. Then ask them what parts of their body are inside. Make a list of them together and see if the children know what each body part does, for example, stomachs break down food. Discuss where their hearts are and ask if anyone knows what hearts do.

After reading

• Take children outside and ask them to hold their hands against their chests. Can they feel their heart beat? Then tell them to run around for five minutes. When they stop, ask them to feel their heart beating in their chest again. What do they notice?

• Make a healthy heart poster together. Put a picture of a heart in the middle and ask each child to draw a picture of food or an activity that is good for our hearts. Stick the children's pictures around the heart and put the poster up in the school.